Parkinson's Tricks

My Story of 20 Years with Parkinsons's Disease

Preface

James Parkinson, born on April 17, 1755, in London/Hoxton, was a versatile scientist who, in addition to his father's profession as a surgeon, conducted research in pharmacy, geology, chemistry, and paleontology and utilized the data he obtained in the field of medicine. Especially through his revolutionary personality, he became known as one of the prominent supporters of the French Revolution while conducting studies in the field of medicine. One of his three published books in the field of medicine, the pamphlet he wrote in 1817 titled "An Essay on the Shaking Palsy," described a neurological disorder that is now referred to as "Parkinson's disease" named after him.

Parkinson's disease, or PD, is a condition that still lacks a fully understood cause and therefore a definitive treatment method, aligning with the saying "it does not kill, nor does it make you laugh." The fact that internationally renowned boxer Muhammad Ali Clay and famous actor Michael J. Fox have been diagnosed with this disease has contributed to its increased recognition. Despite intensive research into the causes, apart from brain trauma, no conclusive findings have been obtained as of this book is being written. Statistical studies have identified events such as gas poisoning and prolonged exposure to heavy metal work as potential causes of the disease.

Bless your health ("geçmiş olsun" in Turkish). This benevolent expression we frequently use in our daily lives is one of the most beautiful wishes that can be said to a friend in a two-word sentence. "Bless your health" and the importance of health as the foundation of everything have been valued throughout history, and the phrase "The people think of wealth and power as the greatest fate, but in this world, a spell of health is the best state." uttered by the significant figure of history, Suleiman the Magnificent, during his illness, has survived until today, emphasizing the significance given to health. As someone who has grasped the importance of health, being a Parkinson's patient, I am honored to share my own interpretations of the effects of this disease on me and the difficulties of living with it, independent of the medical world and the results of scientific research, with my readers.

Diagnosis

1998 fall. In one of my visits to Ankara, where I spent fifteen important years of my life, I find myself in a conversation with friends. I know everyone at the table to some extent. When I meet knowledgeable and well-mannered individuals, I find myself engaged in a high-quality and satisfying conversation.

Among the guests, I am sitting across from a doctor whom I met that night. Due to a need, I got up from the table a few times throughout the night. During my last departure, I noticed his attentive gaze as he carefully watched me until I returned to my seat. I sat down, and at the moment our eyes met, he gestured for me to come closer. To avoid any misunderstanding, we gestured again and I immediately got up and went to him. He wanted me to come close. He told me to visit his office at the hospital tomorrow and emphasized that I must come.

About a month before coming to Ankara, I had noticed that while walking, I wasn't swinging my right arm and my right hand was slightly bent inward with mild spasms. Movements are the actions that occur when the brain's commands are executed. However, the brain never gives direct commands to the limbs. Limbs automatically adjust to the actions the body is supposed to perform. For example, it is very rare to see a healthy person walking without swinging their arms. We cannot say that arm swinging is a command from the brain. Although there are movements that should occur spontaneously without any command, in my case, for example, when walking, I need to focus on walking and swinging my arm to perform this action.

The next day, I am in my doctor friend's office early in the morning. His assistant, told me to wait as she said he would be there shortly. Her timing was accurate. We greeted each other. It was clear from every aspect that he was suffering from the consequences of the previous night. He was quite short, round, and likable. There was a sensory connection with alcohol. The saying "do as the alcoholic doctor says" suited him perfectly. He didn't smoke. While he mentioned the harm of smoking, he never mentioned alcohol as being harmful, as if it were innocent.

He told me that he wanted to perform a brief physical examination and that there might be a possibility of a suspected illness. When I expressed my curiosity, he said, "Hold on. I don't want to say without being certain because it cannot be said that it is a pleasant illness."

"Is it something like a type of cancer?" I asked.

"No," he replied, leaving it at that. Even though he noticed that I was waiting for more information.

He asked me to stand up and extend both of my arms forward, making my fingers tense. I followed his instructions. For about two minutes, with my arms and hands tense, the doctor carefully examined both of my hands. It was as if he was searching for a difference between the two hands.

"You can lower your arms."

I didn't know what was next. He had me perform four more movements. Keeping my hands and arms extended forward, rotating my wrists from side to side. Pulling them backward for balance control and finally tapping the floor with my heel and toe alternately while sitting. After a few simple hand movements and physical examinations, he asked for another doctor, an expert in the field, to come and join us to confirm the findings. After a short conversation with the second doctor, which included many medical terms that I couldn't understand, he had me perform a few more movements similar to the previous ones, seemingly to assess my ability to perform these movements. Lastly, he took me to the corridor to assess my walking pattern. After each movement, perhaps because he was getting closer to an anticipated conclusion, his facial expression became increasingly negative.

The examination was over. I began to wait for the results. The two doctors looked like they agreed after a one-minute discussion. Meanwhile, my gaze was shifting between the two doctors as I wished to receive the results as soon as possible. Their exchange of ideas was brief, and the doctor who arrived later informed me that I would be briefed. The doctor told me to sit down.

Based on the examination they conducted, they informed me that my condition was Parkinson's disease. They explained in detail that my future life could not be planned due to this cursed disease, that Parkinson's progresses insidiously, and there is no treatment method yet found to stop its progression. They emphasized that the disease is not fatal, and as long as I don't develop diseases that may result from the side effects of medications, I could continue living for many years. He provided a detailed explanation. Although he allowed me to ask questions, I didn't have any. I listened while he spoke, but the image of Muhammad Ali didn't leave my mind.

I hadn't done enough research yet. My knowledge about Parkinson's was only superficial, based on the glimpses of Muhammad Ali I saw on television. I only knew that it was an intense trembling disease and slowness of movement that usually occurs in old age.

Thus, in September of 1998, I had the unfortunate encounter with this disease called Parkinson's.

Searching For My Doctor

Treatment is a medical intervention performed through surgery or medication with the aim of eliminating a disease. However, Parkinson's is not a curable disease. The medical world has not reached that stage yet. Medications or surgical interventions only suppress the effects of the disease and provide relief for the patient. Meanwhile, the disease continues to progress underneath.

Although it is a neurological disease, the fact that it is not a disease that every neurologist is interested in was negatively affecting my treatment. In a way that I don't understand even today, I've experienced that doctors may not prefer some patients. Therefore, I embarked on a search for a doctor in Bursa who I could have a good rapport with, someone who would not just stick to their own knowledge, someone I could contact at any time, and perhaps even be a friend. Since then, in Bursa or in Ankara, I have not come across a doctor whom I could say, "This is it." Following a recommendation, I went to a doctor who was an expert in the field of Parkinson's disease, a name I had also heard of. The physical examination, which I had grown tired of repeating each time, began. Then, he sat down at his desk to write a prescription. He started writing. He wrote, and wrote, and wrote... I had conditioned myself to maintain my silence, and I some how succeeded. Just as I was thinking, "That's enough, Selçuk, now intervene," he ran out of space on the prescription, and the medication list seemed to have been tailored accordingly. As the doctor handed me the prescription, he explained that he had written the usage instructions for each medication, such as taking this one before eating and that one after eating. He explained, and I listened.

"Use these medications, and let's see in three months," he said.

"Doctor, I am familiar with most of these medications. Among them, there are interchangeable drugs, and if I were to use them, I don't think I will be alive to come back to you after three months," I said, and I left amidst the doctor's bewildered gaze, without waiting to hear his response. I crumpled the prescription in my hand and threw it into the nearest trash bin.

Following a friend's recommendation, we went to a doctor who had a clinic within Bursa Uludağ University Hospital. The doctor's friendly and talkative demeanor gave me a lot of hope. At first glance, I thought, "This is it," and it was evident from the crowded waiting room that he was an expert in his field. Once again, a familiar physical examination was conducted. To understand me and the condition of my illness, he initiated a conversation, which is something every doctor should do. As he asked questions, I provided answers based on my research findings. Sometimes, I answered before he even asked the next question. I believed that the better a patient describes the difficulties they are experiencing, the easier it becomes to facilitate their treatment. After prescribing one or two medications that I thought could be effective, he told us to come back for a follow-up appointment in fifteen days and escorted us to the door.

The day arrived, and we were at the hospital at the scheduled appointment time. The receptionist told us to wait and informed the doctor of our arrival. A little while later, the doctor came out and approached us, but it seemed as if the person I had initially met during the first examination had disappeared, and a normal and ordinary doctor had taken his place. After the greetings, he said, "Selçuk Bey, I don't consider myself competent enough for your illness and treatment. Please find another doctor for yourself." I suddenly felt like a coach being kicked out of a team. He didn't mean it that way, but that's how I felt. I immediately made a move to leave, in search of another team or teams. The doctor asked, "Are you leaving right away? Won't you ask anything?" He must have been waiting for me to ask the reason for being dismissed. I understood that and decided not to give him the satisfaction of explaining the reason for my dismissal. Unfortunately, I couldn't let go of the courtesy that is a part of my civilized nature.

"I don't have any questions to ask, but if you have something to say, I consider listening to you as one of the important opportunities in my life," I said.

He stared at me for a short while. There was an expression on his face as if he was preparing for a speech on an important topic. I couldn't anticipate that behind this expression, I would see another expression of remorse for fulfilling the obligation he was trying to conceal. He understood that any further delay would put him in a more difficult situation and said the following:

"Selçuk Bey, I don't want to give room for misunderstanding. I'm sure I know more about your illness than you do. But I felt that this knowledge was not enough.

I don't want to waste your time by keeping you occupied. Please excuse me."

I carefully chose my response to prevent this conversation from turning into a polemic.

"Thank you for your openness and sensitivity. I appreciate your care and attention so far," I said as I left the hospital with my wife.

Kids

They grew up with Parkinson's disease since childhood. My youngest son had encountered PH in the womb. My older son, who is six years older, had not grown enough to understand the disease. So, both of them got to know their father and Parkinson's together, they grew up together. In the beginning, it was promising that there were no signs that would negatively affect my daily life. However, the disease had a very insidious nature.

The first five years went by relatively smoothly, despite the negative image of the disease. But after five years, some troublesome things started to happen. I was familiar with the disease. I tried to convince myself not to let it break my courage. I had become my own psychologist. With the support of my family, I considered myself successful in this regard. I still believe in the benefits of therapy, don't get me wrong, and I would recommend it to anyone who is struggling.

I had just started everything. I wouldn't surrender to PD without realizing the life I had envisioned for my family. Among my dreams, providing a suitable environment for my children to receive a quality education had the highest priority. When I talk about education, it's not just about academic education. I needed to work on them becoming exemplary citizens with their behavior and upright stance towards life. Through this, I should be proud of them due to their worldview. I should explain to them that as they build upon their academic education, it is possible to become respectable and rich to the extent they can. I should provide them with the necessary educational environment for them to see that the ways to earn money lie in honest work. In terms of becoming rich in business and self-employment, I am not a positive example. I anticipate that they are inherently equipped with knowledge of how to fail.

I had to do more than my best to ensure that they never lack civic responsibility, both in terms of physical and mental health, and that they reach a level where they can understand the realities of the world. In situations where I fall short, I should try not to reflect it on them as much as possible.

If I have been successful in this regard, I owe a lot to my spouse, who has contributed to every step I have taken.

I can say that the first five years with PH went relatively problem-free or with few issues in terms of symptoms. Every doctor I've seen has confirmed that this disease reacts negatively to stress and distress right away. And there have been moments in my life where I had to go through certain events that prove this idea.

Due to my entrepreneurial nature and the experience and education I gained from my previous work, I didn't see the possibility of my path being blocked. But the developments were prevailing, and I couldn't prevent myself from living with the anxiety of the future. Whenever I tried to act alone and make plans for the future, a hidden hand would block me every time. Despite everything, time, which never changes its speed, was calling me to be rational.

I didn't take into account the power of the enemy within me, which would not forgive me for trying to be heroic. I was like Don Quixote, unable to see the power difference when attacking windmills.

Work

During the years I met PD, I was still continuing with my normal work life. The rate of obstruction in my life and work was around 20%. My job was not easy at all. On the surface, I was the partner, and actually the owner of the construction company that my brother and I had established three years ago. While I was trying to reduce the impact of the disease, I couldn't cope with the stress that had a negative effect.

The company's founding philosophy required both of us to know one thing very well: the need for division of tasks. There was no need to discuss how it would be done. As accepted by himself, I was responsible for technical issues and construction site organization. Naturally, it was clear who would be responsible for which area. My successful track record in construction site organization, which was known by those close to me and also by my brother, was already well-established. In fact, the logic behind both his proposal and my acceptance was that I would fill his gap in this regard. However, this thought alone was not a sufficient reason for me in this partnership, of course. There were certain things that I found lacking in myself, and my brother had some abilities that could compensate for those shortcomings. We didn't have to spend very long periods of time. I didn't have a clear idea about it because I didn't follow the business life closely. But that was the image he left on me.

To some extent, I can say that I saw the validity of this idea. With the limited company we established, we achieved successful projects, although not as much as my dreams and expectations. I take pride in saying that both of us made the right decisions and reached success under equal conditions.

During the early days of working on our company, we faced many challenges. My most important goal for this company was its growth. Until that day, my brother, who had been struggling alone, unfortunately made some wrong practices and took on projects using files belonging to others. Even though this could bring in money, growth was not possible in this way. I strived for the company to have ideals and principles, to become a corporate firm capable of achieving great things. However, my brother's understanding of partnership gradually revealed itself and my dreams about the company remained beyond reach.

Initially, we produced good results with this partnership. The consequences of forming a good duo were apparent, albeit with some difficulties. My brother's understanding of business and partnership negatively affected our work and dampened my enthusiasm. It became an increasingly distressing situation. The partnership relationship that was normal when I was present was being discussed in different ways in my absence. The arguments had escalated to the point of being topics of discussion in family gatherings, which came as the biggest surprise of my life.

Deep brain stimulation (DBS) and Speech Problems

After the DBS surgery, I couldn't prevent the damage caused by these and similar incidents that stressed me out. The doctor who performed the DBS operation himself was left in the dust. Shortly after the surgery, he referred me to another doctor for battery adjustment. I frequently visited this doctor because the battery adjustment process is not completed in a single visit. I met with this doctor frequently.

Meanwhile, Doctor Cenk Akbostancı, who adjusted the battery after the surgery for the voice and speech, or rather the inability to speak problem, recommended a specialized treatment expert. I made an appointment on the same day and went to the place located in a luxurious apartment in Çankaya. Since my wife had some business to attend to, she dropped me off there and left, saying she would return in half an hour.

When it was my turn, I entered the doctor's office with an assistant. The doctor or treatment expert was a natural blonde woman in her mid-thirties to early forties. Whether she was beautiful, charming, pleasant, attractive, or had a bit of each, I still can't decide even today. After a brief introduction, she got up from her desk and sat in the chair across from me.

"Mr. Selçuk, your speech is gradually diminishing due to Parkinson's disease. Preventing it is up to you. You will need to perform the mouth and tongue movements I'm going to show you at frequent intervals," she said. She asked if I was ready.

"I'm ready," I said.

"I didn't hear you."

She wanted me to raise my voice a little more. As loudly as possible, I said, "I'm ready."

Not finding my tone sufficient, she accompanied it with a few stretching exercises to increase my voice. She asked me to make sounds. This exercise lasted for about ten minutes. At that moment, I saw the benefits of this exercise.

Next, it was time for tongue movements for clear pronunciation of words. That's when the film broke for me. The distance between us was no more than thirty centimeters. She wanted me to extend my tongue as far as possible and move it in a circular motion as if making a loop in the air to activate my seemingly motionless tongue. She wanted me to do the same movement at the same time. After each tongue movement, she asked me to speak, which made me realize the benefits of this movement. The tongue movements proved to be helpful. However, inadvertently, my thoughts took an unexpected turn. The tongue movements had to end as soon as possible, but I didn't want them to. Suddenly, she stood up, saying, "See you tomorrow at the same time, Mr. Selçuk. You may leave now. Just retract your tongue before you leave, please." I cannot remember ever feeling so embarrassed in my life.

I didn't go back, using the excuse of it being expensive. In fact, I cannot explain how much I wanted to go there. I didn't go because I knew I shouldn't. It is said that I have high self-confidence in my surroundings, but this time, I couldn't trust myself. I would practice the tongue movements she showed me in front of the mirror but couldn't succeed. I would mix up the order of the movements and sometimes realize that I had left the movement incomplete. It was only the impact she left on me during that session.

Am I unfair in not going back?

Tricks

My spouse and I had acquired enough knowledge about PD. Now, our next step was to conduct research on alternative treatments that could be effective against this incurable disease, along with medication and surgical treatment methods to find ways to delay its progression. During the first five years, I was able to manage my work, my spouse, and my children without disrupting my normal life and without losing much of my quality of life.

Of course, this doesn't mean that the five-year period passed without feeling the effects of the illness. The progression rate of PD is similar to that of a tree's growth. No matter how closely you observe, you cannot see a tree growing in the blink of an eye. But one day, you notice that it has grown. The progression rate of PD can vary from patient to patient. This aspect of progression fascinated me the most. After realizing this difference, I was able to find ways to improve my quality of life or at least maintain it at satisfactory levels. I never felt the need to conduct research on this matter. If my living conditions were causing the symptoms of PD to become more pronounced, and I noticed it, I made efforts to change my living conditions to the extent that my strength and intellect allowed, and I mostly achieved positive results. However, it attracted my attention that the doctors' approach to this issue was just plain advice. I've never heard from a doctor that the effect of sleep deprivation on PD is so important. An important detail that should not be forgotten here is that an extra hour or two of arbitrary sleep after waking up gave more negative results than insomnia. Nothing more, no less. The recipe for quality and timely sleep is spontaneous awakening sleep without external influences. Let's never forget that.

I never experienced tremors, which are common in most PD patients. The most significant difficulties for me were slowness of movement and walking. The years between 2005 and 2008 were particularly challenging, as this problem reached an unbearable stage.

We accelerated our research on PH with the help of the internet. At the American Hospital in Istanbul, we found a potential solution by targeting the relevant area in the brain to reduce the effects of PD through burning, which seemed like a way to delay the progression of the disease by a few years. Shortly thereafter, we came across another surgical solution called Deep Brain Stimulation (DBS), performed by the same doctor in the same place, which we opted for after conducting numerous research and watching videos of the surgery. My spouse and I made the decision together. We identified three doctors who performed this operation. We made an appointment with a doctor in Izmir and traveled there.

Broad Beans

It is worth mentioning the broad beans, which is commonly used in many medications and contains dopamine. During the early days, another doctor who was monitoring my condition at Cerrahpaşa Hospital, advised me to eat broad bean stew without yogurt as an additive, as long as it wasn't excessive. In the next check-up, his first question was whether I had tried the broad bean stew. My response brought a smile to his face.

"I couldn't remember whether it was broad beans or okra, so I didn't try it."

Before we set off for Izmir, my spouse prepared a jar of olive oil-based broad beans to bring along. Our journey to Izmir was quite challenging. Except for the PD tremors, all the effects had intensified. Walking, in particular, was extremely difficult. To avoid being late for the doctor's appointment, we left the hotel early. Although the doctor's office wasn't far, even a single step felt distant to me. Each step I took had a significant emotional cost.

Especially, I couldn't lift my right leg. In fact, instead of my leg carrying me, I was carrying it. Instead of lifting my foot and moving it forward about 20-30 cm, as it should be, my foot and its accomplice, my leg, were stubbornly resisting like a stubborn donkey to cross the bridge. Breaking its resistance meant liberation from this disease. What could be called walking in theory was actually a crawling-like movement. We started our journey with extremely tiny steps that represented a step further than crawling. I made progress with each step, covering about 1/10th of a normal step's distance. There was no name for this way of walking, but I had given it a measurement unit: the centimeter-based walking pace.

It is impossible for me to divert my attention to another subject besides walking. While walking, or if we can call it walking, you have to focus solely on walking. Feet that are already reluctant to move take any opportunity and excuse to change the focus of your attention, and they completely give up on walking. They almost wanted to walk backward.

Speaking of... I wondered how it would be to try walking backward? I wanted to stop and calm down, and I wanted to try going backward. I stop. Taking a breath and stepping back with my left foot, lightly touching the tip of my toes to the ground, I can then move my left foot forward and take the challenging forward step. This way, I easily cover the distance of six steps to the building's door, then three steps to the elevator. I'm happy for successfully taking these three steps using this new method. However, moving my feet is quite exhausting. After all, I was the one carrying my feet, which are supposed to carry me. At this pace, even reaching the appointment on time becomes a risk. We reached the building's door. At that moment, we greeted a gentleman who wanted to pass us. Judging by his appearance, he seemed to be a well-dressed gentleman. So, not everything is about appearances. The man doesn't even offer his help. I wanted to say "what a jerk" but kept it to myself. We manage to knock on the door through an adventurous endeavor. A helpful lady opens the door and brings a wheelchair in a rush, probably finding whatever she saw in my and my wife's appearance. With the help of others, I manage to sit in the wheelchair, although it's difficult. Among the melancholic gazes of the patients and their families waiting in the waiting room, I take a few centimeter-sized steps to the designated waiting chair and manage to sit with the assistance of others.

This challenging walk has given me something. By pretending to take a step back, I can move my other foot forward. Somehow, I can control my leg through a trick. It's not a small gain; perhaps there are a few more movements like this. By trial and error, it might be possible to improve my walking quality at least to some extent.

After resting for a few minutes, my wife opens a small jar from her bag and takes a disgusting bean from it. It was evident that she had put a lot of effort into making it edible. I close my eyes and only take two bites with a fork. Five minutes later, when I tell my wife that I need to go to the bathroom, she quickly gets up to get the wheelchair. However, something very frightening happens while we wait for the device. I had managed to stand up without any assistance and walked from one end of the room to the other. What could be scarier than that? I believe I'm dead, but at that moment, some small events prove that I'm not dead. The same fear and astonishment turn the patients in the room into motionless robots. This show ends with my wife's explanation. Fresh beans, a plant or vegetable that temporarily relieves me and compensates for the lack of dopamine in my brain. Does my wife have some kind of special talent? Or was it just a coincidence? When the dosage problem of bean treatment is resolved, this illness will be a thing of the past. It's all about fresh beans, not medication or surgery. Hooray for fresh beans! The waiting patients lined to get the recipe from my wife. My wife is equally surprised.

However, despite repeated attempts, we couldn't quite find the right dosage for the beans. There was no room for mistakes in dosage adjustment. If it's insufficient, it has no effect; if it's excessive, it causes chaos in the brain. Sometimes, we continue these experiments when it's bean season. It wouldn't be accurate to say that I don't get any results. Doctors haven't reached a common concnlusion on this matter. The reason is that the active ingredient in the medication is already derived from beans. Therefore, it is considered more appropriate by most doctors not to use it because adjusting the dosage is difficult.

The Young Doctor

Since my medication report has expired, I need to renew it, and it has to be done by a specialist doctor. We wait for an appointment at the Neurology clinic in the State Hospital. When my name appears on the screen, with the support of my wife, I stand up and was about to enter through the open door for the examination when, despite preparing myself very well for entering and exiting narrow places and doors, experiencing freezing, what I call the freezing phenomenon, becomes inevitable most of the time. In front of me, there is a doctor who can be the best example of the young doctor category with his physique that appears to be in his late twenties or early thirties. As I struggled to take one more step from the door sill, he spoke to me from where he was sitting in a soft and soothing voice, "Could you please stop there without trying to enter? Now, calm down. Before taking a step, stroke your hair with one hand. Meanwhile, let entering be your goal."

My hair is too short to be combed with a hand, but I understood what he wanted from me. I did as he said and sat in the chair across from him. As I mentioned earlier, I had found a method where I could take a forward step by pretending to step my toes backward when trying to walk. The hand gesture that allowed me to sit in front of him was a Parkinson's trick that I hadn't yet realized.

Within the limited examination time with the young doctor, we had a positive conversation about Parkinson's tricks. He told me that I should replicate these physical movements, which we refer to as tricks, that I should constantly make attempts to discover and uncover these movements, and that the movement is amplified by breathing support. I feel like he must have experienced what I have been going through. Otherwise, how could he know these things without experiencing them? I don't think medical books contain information about Parkinson's tricks and similar techniques. When I struggled to take a step, the only solution offered by doctors was to extend their feet in front of me to help me overcome an obstacle. However, I had already tried this action of overcoming the obstacle in front. My Parkinson's didn't fall for that trick.

I liked this young doctor. I can say that I didn't see his behavior in every doctor. He mentioned that he wanted to become a Parkinson's specialist during our conversation. I wish him success on this path.

First Surgery

If we return to İzmir, the secretary lady, like the other guests in the waiting room, witnessed the incident with a bewildered look. However, it was expected that she would be accustomed to all kinds of patients. As soon as she informed the doctor about what she saw, we were called into the doctor's office amidst the astonished gazes of the patient and their family members. I recognize him when I see him. It turns out that our doctor, whom I just passed by and burnt his ears, was our doctor. He saw us but didn't intervene because he thought it would be wrong to interfere in this situation. Although he did not have a different opinion on the broad beans, he said that it makes sense to continue experimenting with it, on season, and with small amounts.

To provide information about the DBS operation, which is our main topic, he started explaining on a device he took out of the drawer. This device is a matchbox-sized device manufactured with high technology, which can work for 4-6 years depending on usage, and is nothing more than a special battery. This device is implanted under the skin in a region on the right breast of the body. From there, it is connected to two special metal rods that extend from the depths of the brain through two openings made in the center of the skull, using special cables that run under the skin. The adjustment of the battery is done by a specialized doctor after the operation is completed.

This procedure was relatively new. Therefore, the Ministry of Health had not yet adapted to this process. The cost of the procedure reached figures that could not be compared to an ordinary surgery, and it was unthinkable for me to cover this money. Doctor emphasized the need for the regulation in the law to be realized as soon as possible and said goodbye. With the conviction that my missing information about DBS has been completed, we left.

I continued my search in Ankara. We are with the second doctor who performs DBS surgeries. This person is someone whose father once served as the President of the Constitutional Court, and he is a name I deeply respect.

In addition to the cost covered by social security for the surgery, we agree to pay an additional 26,000 Turkish Lira (~20,000 USD at the time) for all expenses. We set a date for the surgery. On the designated day, I am admitted to the hospital.

Surgery Day

My first visitor is the barber. My hair needs to be shaved. As a result, preparations are completed, and to initiate the surgery, a thick circular sectioned ring is placed around my forehead with four screws (mercilessly) tightened. In my opinion, this is the most difficult and painful part of the surgery. I am fixed like a material ready for machining, firmly fastened to the operating table with the same ring. There are 10 people in the room: a doctor instructing the staff, a representative from the battery company, the surgeon, and other assistants. Everyone knows their job. My doctor also joins the team. As local anesthesia is injected into my skull for the purpose of local numbing, the second pain I feel after the screws is this. After the local anesthesia, I am unaware of the events happening around my head. At one point, I heard the sound of a drill. I knew that my skull was being pierced, but I didn't feel anything. I realize that the procedure has started thanks to the sound the drill makes as it penetrates my skull. I was unaware of what was happening to my head since no sound was coming from the remaining procedures. With this two-hour operation, the electrodes are delicately placed in the depths of my brain, which were previously determined through some calculations and leave no room for error, through the openings made in the skull. Thus, the first stage of the surgery is completed. The next morning, I undergo the second stage of the operation. This time, I am put to sleep. The procedure is completed with the connection made from the battery implanted under the right breast, under the skin, to the electrodes in my head, which are again routed under the skin.

A two-day marathon comes to an end.

An amazing result.

It's a miracle. An incredible event. The pre-surgery troubles have ended, and I now better understand the meaning of being reborn into the world. I am amazed at having regained my health before the disease. I think about how I can thank the invisible heroes who provided me with this happiness, especially the ones who invented this battery and my doctor, and others who made this operation possible in Türkiye. A simple thank you should not be enough of what they have done. I can't care about the money I paid. I will be grateful to them for the rest of my life.

We had a meeting with the doctor to discuss my future life without the dependence on medication from the hospital. Some things he said seemed interesting to me. While I was taking in his necessary opinions, the doctor continued with his routine explanations. One of his advice caught my attention:

"At least for a year, postpone your important decisions, even if they seem unreasonable. Do not make significant commitments."

Confidence

Physically, I am healthy as I was before the illness. But I haven't forgotten what I went through. Even if I wanted to forget, I couldn't. With every movement, I remember the past. Any physical movement I wasn't able to perform before the surgery, now feels like a huge achievement.

I sense that the change is not only physical. I noticed that I understand people better and make more accurate judgments about individuals compared to before. I acted with utmost certainty in every decision. It seemed like I had become a bit cruel. I started to sense dissatisfaction in the people around me, especially in my close friendships. But in every matter, I was right, and my decision was the correct one. This selfishness was disturbing my close relatives, friends, and even my family. But no one could claim that I was wrong. The discomfort people felt around me had reached an extent where they contacted the doctor and complained about the consequences of this operation.

The doctor, who was experienced in this matter, had a very logical response to such complaints. He said, "We played with the man's brain. You must get used to this change in behavior." It was clear that what the doctor meant was not fully understood. After a new complaint, the doctor put an end to the conversation.

"If there is a change, it means it's a positive change."

What the doctor meant was, take care of yourself. After a long hiatus, I decided to return to work. I had left the company. I would work alone or collaborate on a project basis. I packed my bag and set off. I had no doubts about success. I had a strong problem-solving ability within me. There was no unsolvable problem or impossible task for me. My self-confidence was at its peak.

Reality

It didn't take long for such exaggerated self-assurance to collide with the realities of life. The negativity started with a speech disorder. I realized that I had difficulty speaking. My voice would fade, words would get tangled on my tongue, and I couldn't say what I wanted to say. Moreover, this malfunction progressed rapidly.

Around that time, a job opportunity emerged. General Directorate of Natural Disasters had initiated a project to build new disaster-resistant housing in areas at risk of natural disasters such as floods, avalanches, landslides, and rockfalls. However, due to slow bureaucracy and the government's financial constraints, there had been no progress for twenty years. The claimants had almost forgotten about the issue. Using some of my connections, I managed to bring the files to light. The government, under the name "Assistance for Building Homes" (EYY), committed to depositing a certain amount per household into the bank accounts of eligible claimants in exchange for their entitlements. The claimants were free to choose a contractor of their own selection, under the technical supervision of the Ministry of Public Works.

I set out with a friend from that region in Bursa. We picked up a person from Ankara who had experience in these matters. Our goal was to persuade the claimants and make contracts for the construction of 27 disaster-resistant houses in a village. This way, we would secure a project worth one million lira (~650.000 USD at the time), which was not difficult to execute and required serial production. Thanks to my colleague from Ankara, who had previously established relationships with the claimants, we got acquainted with important figures, starting with the village headman. With his efforts, we obtained power of attorney from the claimants to carry out the construction and to pay their entitled remunerations into their accounts. We brought the notary to the village to complete this procedure. We mingled with the claimants and their families, gathering in the village square. We managed to combine work and entertainment.

I was at the helm of a job that required meeting people, establishing new connections, and forming social relationships, but I couldn't accomplish that. Being unable to speak was mentally devastating for me. It was very difficult to explain this to people. After a while, as a second surprise, balance problems began to emerge, and I reached a point where I couldn't walk without assistance. Unexpected falls started to occur out of nowhere. While walking, suddenly, my legs would freeze, like a car coming to a stop. While my legs stopped, the upper part of my body, from the waist up, wanted to continue walking without any connection. The result was evident. I don't know how long my knees could endure these falls, but it was clear that my PD was starting to take effect again.

Meanwhile, a stroke of misfortune found me. The project for which I had made contracts came under the control of the Provincial Special Administration, i.e., the governorship, within the Ministry of Public Works. The contract texts and power of attorney documents instantly became invalid. Everything had to be started over. Instead of the Ministry of Public Works, the Provincial Special Administration requested that "Provincial Special Administration" be written in the contract and power of attorney documents. Although proposals for new powers of attorney on behalf of the governorship had been submitted by the claimants, I lacked the financial and physical strength to start everything from scratch. This chapter closed with losses. The money I used as capital support also has put the supporting parties in a difficult situation. I am facing difficulties in repaying this money, even to this day.

As the years go by, looking back to appreciate the previous year and realizing that I was making a move last year that I couldn't make today, it depresses me. Parkinson's disease continues to progress. Compared to the previous year, PD slowly progresses with classic symptoms such as freezing, slowed movement, and balance impairment, and new symptoms emerge. Speech impairment becomes an inability to speak, taking a step further. I prepare myself to speak, mentally rehearse, fully focus on speaking, and start talking. However, I struggle to complete the third word.

Talking Again

But one morning, I woke up and realized that I could speak. I was very happy when I realised this. I regained my ability to speak. It was very important to me. With this morale, I felt like I could overcome Parkinson's.

I used to believe in miracles, but I never relied on miracles in my life. It didn't take me long to learn the scientific facts. The conductive diodes implanted in the brain must pass through the speech center or its influence area in order to reach the targeted area. When energy is supplied to the electrodes, the voice becomes softer and the ability to speak is lost. Conversely, when the energy current is somehow cut off, I instantly regain my natural voice tone without any seconds lost. I notice this with the third depleted battery. But without the battery, Parkinson's couldn't be managed. And the third battery was installed. The three and a half years I spent with the third battery were challenging in terms of speech, but I managed. During my last appointment for replacement (4th Battery), the doctor, using a control device reserved for doctors, measured the remaining battery level and told me that the battery was about to run out. Due to the examination requirement, the battery that was already about to run out was disabled with the control device available only to doctors.

When the battery was stopped or depleted, I strangely started feeling better. Walking and balance were great. My speech was fantastic, with a perfect tone. It was never said that this battery would cure me anyway, the main aim was syptom relief. I knew my happiness wouldn't last. Still, I believe that discovering something new would be beneficial for me.

In 2007, when I first encountered the DBS operation, before it was applied to my body, I asked the doctor who introduced me to the device about a question regarding the device. He didn't know. He said I should ask the question to the representative of the importing company. He might be right. The doctor couldn't know how this battery was made with what kind of technology. A remote control programmed to turn the battery on and off is given to the patient's family members. According to the information I received, this remote control has never been used by any patient so far. The importing company, on the other hand, didn't provide any training to the patient or their family members about this remote control because if the patient could use this device, it would result in a significant loss in sales volume. It was not possible to get an answer to the question of whether the device could be turned on and off multiple times (for example, three times a day).

By a simple calculation, keeping the battery on for 1/3 of the day and off for the rest would save significant battery life. Therefore, I decided to use the recently installed battery in this way. I can confidently say that this method was not only for saving purposes. The benefit of DBS without medication is around 10-15%. I never experienced tremors at any stage of the disease. My observations indicated that DBS was highly effective, around 90%, for patients with tremors.

I was late. The employee of the company I mentioned earlier didn't provide me with the necessary explanation due to the well-known reason. I don't blame them because I used to work as a salesperson, so I understand. They didn't even tell me that this battery can be used in an on-off manner like they do when needed. Currently, I have been using the 4th battery for approximately 6 months, opening and closing it about twice a day on average. When I open the battery, it feels like receiving a powerful punch. This punch lasts for about three seconds, and after three seconds, there is a sense of relief in the legs, and the body gains better mobility than when the battery is closed. When the battery is on, the difficulty of taking steps (freezing) is resolved, but the steps become shorter. Balance issues arise, and walking without assistance or support becomes challenging. It's difficult to answer whether I have a battery or not. The fact that the necessary electrical installation was done in my body during the first surgery makes it harder for me to answer this question. My ability to speak becomes more difficult during battery usage. The freezing problem in my foot disappears when I drive. Each of the previous three batteries had a lifespan of around 3.5 years, so it is possible to determine how many years it will last with this economical usage through a simple calculation. The proof of my claim will only be visible when this battery runs out.

(Note: This battery is still in use in its 5th year, 2023)

The first battery replacement caused me a lot of distress. The excitement and anxiety were mixed, just like everything else that is the first.

Healthcare Workers

On April 20, 2012, the transition into summer is intensely felt. I am in Ankara, and today a sandstorm of unprecedented magnitude is wreaking havoc on the capital city. I am caught in this storm, which can be called unprecedented in the history of Ankara, the moment I enter the hospital room where I will spend about fifteen days. In other words, I'm inside. Being inside doesn't prevent me from feeling the intensity of the storm; on the contrary, as soon as I enter, the upper opening parts of the windows, poorly constructed, fully open, bringing the storm inside. Already, experiencing the excitement and apprehension of being admitted to the hospital, this incident makes me wonder, "Where have we come to?" I reassure myself that there is no need to panic and maintain my composure as usual, and I start closing the windows with all my strength. While doing this task, I am annoyed by the poor quality of the windows' construction. Soon, clarity replaces my anger. Because I am well aware that these jobs are carried out through public tender, awarded to the lowest bidder, which is a flawed method. It's very easy to blame the contractor or the person, but one should not forget the fact that the main culprit is the institution approving these impossible physical tasks to be done at low prices. This natural event, which lasts about an hour, ends without turning into a real disaster, and everything calms down. I arrange my belongings, and apart from the room cleaner, no one comes and goes for about half an hour. I try to rest in a semi-sitting position, utilizing the feature of my bed that can be adjusted according to my preference.

My mind is in a state of confusion. The battery that I have been carrying in my body for three and a half years to significantly reduce the effects of Parkinson's disease is about to run out. Should I have gotten this procedure done by the person who performed the first operation? Of course, that was my initial preference. However, even though the social security institution covers the cost of the battery, the fee they demanded exceeded my means. That's why I am here, at this government hospital. Moreover, this hospital was known as the worst hospital in Ankara. Financial hardship was the main concern, and I had to have the procedure done here.

Fortunately, my doctor, Selçuk Bey, whom I met a few days ago and who happens to share my name, is the head of this department and a dedicated individual. His genuine and warm behavior towards his patients clearly shows his passion for his profession. It is unthinkable otherwise, as one cannot understand the nature of being a doctor without being a patient and having close contact with them. In recent years, I have been fortunate enough to have this opportunity. Although my chance came as a result of an unfortunate event, it made me realize that viewing doctors as mere merchants or engineers would be wrong. Above all, the genuine love for humanity they carry within them enables them to enjoy their work.

Unfortunately, I had learned quite late that April 18, 2012, was a dark day for doctors. Two days ago, the incident in the city of Gaziantep had left the doctors in a somber state. The black ribbons worn by all hospital staff members around their collars and the black-and-white ID photo of a young doctor symbolized intense protest and mourning. In Gaziantep, a lunatic had held the young doctor responsible for the death of his eighty-five-year-old cancer-stricken grandfather on the operating table and had stabbed and killed him. Posters condemning this shameful incident were hung on every door in the hospital, and the doctors had planned various actions for that day and the following day. This situation had deeply embarrassed me, as if I were a representative of the opposing side.

Whether they are doctors working in healthcare institutions or not, I would have liked to apologize as a patient to everyone, from caregivers to nurses, drivers to janitors. There was something else I wanted to express. You may think of me as a revengeful barbarian, but I could not refrain from expressing myself. The name of this monster was being kept secret by the press. I hoped this name becomes known, and all doctors took note of it in a place they will never forget. They should take note so that one day, when this monster comes to their doorstep, they treat him the way he deserved.

However, as much as I desired such a thing, I am absolutely certain that doctors, who are among the few who remain loyal to their professional oaths, would not do that.

I sincerely wish patience and rationality to the entire healthcare community, who cannot tolerate the recurrence of such events, and I hope that the protests that have taken place after this incident will be in accordance with the dignity of their sacred profession. Because that is what suits them. It should never be forgotten that there is no person who has never passed by a doctor at least once in their lifetime.

Compared to other countries, Turkish citizens encounter government officials more frequently, and their interaction with them never seems to end. Turkish citizens have long been in a subservient position in the face of government officials. The dominance of officials over citizens has persisted for many years, and to some extent, it still continues. In recent years, with the increase in the education level of government employees and the support of civil society organizations such as consumer rights, as well as the rise of civic awareness among citizens, the dialogue between the counter and front of the desk has softened, and commanding officials have turned into requesting ones. This is particularly evident in the police force, especially in traffic. However, the situation is slightly different in the healthcare sector. The relationship between citizens and healthcare professionals takes on a different dimension when it involves human life. The majority of doctors, who have received the highest level of academic education, have integrated the consciousness of treating humans as humans into their academic training. Love for humanity should be at the forefront. Otherwise, would it be possible for them to continue this profession tirelessly?

On the part of the citizens, the situation seems to be completely opposite. The class of citizens that doctors dealing with in state healthcare institutions is more unaware. For them, what matters is their own patient, and the doctor's duty is to heal them without any excuses. As if the doctor is a magician, and the patient's fate is at their fingertips.

One of the beds in the two-bed room is empty. I learn from the caregiver that an 18-year-old youth who is being admitted today will come to the bed next to mine. I have difficulty sleeping on the first night. It's already 3:00 a.m. and I still haven't slept. I look out the window. Although it's the same view I've been looking at all day, it looks very different at night. The first thing that catches the eye when looking out the window is the entrance to the emergency department. This scene, which is quite lively after midnight, is where the final point is put to violent incidents. Patients who arrive as a result of ordinary injuries, sudden illnesses, or traffic accidents until a certain hour of the night are all forensic cases after 3:00 a.m. The cluster of events that unfolds like the final scene of a different story every night can be a rich content for a novelist. Everything is calm before the movie starts. It has never been a surprise that this calmness signifies the silence before the storm. While calmness prevails here, a fight may have started in an unseen place, knives may have been drawn, and guns may have been fired.

The interesting part is that incidents that seem to have been scheduled for 3:00 a.m. start in the hospital emergency department with a plus or minus ten-minute difference. The injuries usually occur with a knife, and the angry relatives or supporters of the injured party make things difficult for the healthcare professionals by venting their anger. It is not unlikely for the three police officers who are on duty constantly to join the reinforcement force without delay when necessary.

Another trouble in the emergency department is intoxicated injured individuals or their relatives. They don't understand what is being said. While trying to bring the injured person to the emergency department, they are chased by the enemy all the way to the hospital door. Suddenly, chaos breaks out. The intervention of the additional police force puts an end to the situation. Another frequently repeated incident is the death of a person who came to the emergency department due to a fight or illness because the intervention was insufficient. It's as if doomsday is happening. The relatives of the deceased start screaming, running around, breaking windows and frames, kicking the surrounding objects, in short, causing a commotion. The magnitude of their pain does not justify their actions. I don't think that when a patient who has a chance of surviving enters the emergency department, they have the right to harm others when they learn about the death news from inside. This chaos and disturbing situation sometimes last until daylight.

Medical education is a lifelong process that involves simultaneously experiencing theory and practice. It is a difficult, challenging, and patience-requiring profession. If there is any sacred profession, it is undoubtedly the most sacred profession in the world. The most demanding aspect of this profession is the dialogue with patients and their families. Doctors may be tired but not discouraged. They are prepared to sacrifice day and night to bring relief to their patients. All they need is a little understanding and trust. The exhaustion never crosses the mind of the patient's family. They are agitated and aggressive. At that moment, these two parties, who seem like a lit match and gunpowder, will continue to need each other as long as life goes on. Especially the patient should know that the need for a doctor will never cease.

Side Effects

Reducing the daily dosage of PD medication is crucial in terms of side effects. PD itself is not fatal, meaning it is not the cause of death. However, the side effects of high-dose medication taken over many years often lead to death due to kidney failure. The fewer pills taken, the less affected one is by the side effects. Currently, the aim of research in this field is to develop medication that can be taken once every twenty-four hours with minimized side effects.

PD is a brain disease, and the brain is the most vital organ defining human beings. Even if the remaining parts of a person whose brain death has occurred are flawless and healthy, they can only be of use to another patient with a healthy brain through organ donation.

PD medications are drugs that provide the missing dopamine substance to the brain caused by its depletion. However, delivering this substance to the relevant area is the most significant challenge in treating Parkinson's disease. This is partly achieved by using additional medications in conjunction with dopamine-containing drugs. However, these auxiliary medications have some non-physiological side effects, such as disturbances in personal behavior, gambling addiction, and increased sexual impulses. In particular, the uncontrollable increase in sexual impulses can lead to significant problems between the patient and their spouse. However, a conscious patient's spouse can resolve this issue by seeing it as a result of the disease. As long as medication use continues, this problem usually persists and causes major issues between spouses. The reason for this problem is that the increase in sexual desire is only in the brain, and physically, it often conflicts with the thoughts of an elderly and tired body.

Years ago, during the initial stages of PD, I met a patient from the southeast region over the phone. He would call me approximately every fifteen days. He would ask for information about PH and request that I recommend a doctor. He was about ten years older than me. He would say that I was very helpful to him and value my advice. Our last conversation was five years ago, and during that conversation, he said he wanted to tell me something about PD but was embarrassed. I immediately understood and told him that some medications could cause it. A week later, he called again and said his wife had gone to her father's house, meaning she had run away. That was our last conversation unless he calls me again in the future.

Another problem is constipation. Despite claims that it is related to the variety of foods consumed, the problem continues regardless of what I eat. This problem, which varies from person to person, must be solved without a doubt. If not resolved, there is a possibility of diseases related to the digestive system such as colon cancer.

Gas

PD. I understand it doesn't suit me, and it doesn't look good on me. But it is not a disease that exists because of my request, and it will not go away if I tell it to go away. I don't listen to nonsense like destiny, fate, it was meant to be, everything is from God...

By thoroughly examining my experiences and conducting retrospective research, I am trying to find the real and scientific causes of the disease. While doing this, without any data in hand, I compare the incidents that could potentially cause PD among my past experiences with other probable causes. Around 1987, I took on a job for myself based on an offer from a hydroelectric power plant construction project in Niksar, a district of Tokat. The job was to open an 8000-meter-long circular section tunnel with a diameter of 3.8 meters, starting from a dam (Almus Dam) located behind the high mountains with dense fog across from Niksar, and to incorporate the water of the dam into the system as electrical energy generated due to the region's geological structure. My job was to manufacture the tunnel formwork that covers the surface of this tunnel with concrete and deliver it in a functional state. The system I was going to manufacture needed to be able to perform 12 meters of tunnel concrete lining in 24 hours. I had committed to performing the general maintenance and repair of the formwork during any breakdown or malfunction, and to ensure that any kind of malfunction is promptly resolved by me until the completion of the tunnel, with the condition of being paid for the service. Within three months, I completed the production of the tunnel formwork, which weighs 12 tons and would work according to the specifications, and ensured the start of the project.

One evening, after dinner, I was lying on the couch watching television to relax after a long day. The news started, and the first news story captivated my attention. I found it hard to breathe. I couldn't believe what I was hearing. According to the news, during the concrete pouring process in a tunnel under construction in Tokat/Niksar, a gas leak occurred that was not detectable by the senses but caused instant death with a single breath, resulting in the loss of 18 lives. It was a complete disaster.

According to the subsequent accounts, 12 people involved in the concrete work inside the tunnel could not be reached after a while. When the concrete mixer truck that transported concrete into the tunnel did not return within a reasonable time, panic broke out outside. There was a telephone system set up for communication, but despite numerous attempts, no one answered. The panic outside intensified. There were 12 people inside the tunnel who couldn't be reached. I knew most of these people, including a few who were from the same family. A group of five people consisting of those who couldn't get any news from their son, without thinking about the consequences, rushed into the tunnel by climbing onto the bucket of a rubber-wheeled loader that happened to be there. Normally, it would take 15 minutes to reach the tunnel. They couldn't be reached for 45 minutes. With a single breath of the gas inside, there was no need for a second breath. According to the accounts of those who witnessed the scene, the driver of the loader was found holding onto the steering wheel. What followed contained extremely dramatic scenes. These were unbelievable sights. The nature of such an effective gas, which took 18 lives, was understood at the end of the research period.

Three months ago, after the tunnel drilling was completed, the airflow from both ends made the work difficult, so the unused end was sealed with old logs found in the vicinity. Thus, the cold airflow that affected the work was eliminated. A week before this incident, those dry logs inexplicably started to burn. The people in the vicinity saw the fire and extinguished it with a few buckets of water. Since the logs were not completely burned, no further action was taken, and the incident was forgotten as an instant event. The logs, which appeared to be completely extinguished, actually emitted a kind of gas that was invisible, odorless, and astonishingly, did not show any signs of poisoning such as dizziness or nausea, and it silently approached the opposite end of the closed mouth of the tunnel like a monster swallowing everyone in its path. And inevitably, a disaster occurred.

A month passed since the incident. I received the news. Work would resume in the tunnel, and I was called to perform the maintenance and restore the tunnel formwork, covered by the paid guarantee, the condition of which was unknown after the incident. The next day, in the office of the construction site manager, four people responsible for opening the tunnel, including me, five people in total, under the management of the construction site manager, were making a detailed plan. The first priority was safety.

This was going to be the first time entering the tunnel after the accident. After determining that the incident was caused by a fire, the burning logs were removed, and the tunnel was left open at both ends for three days. This should have allowed it to be cleared of toxic gases thanks to the resulting air circulation. As a precaution after the accident, work was halted, and entry to the tunnel was sealed by authorized organizations. Thus, we proceeded with confidence that the tunnel has been completely cleaned. We entered the tunnel on foot along with four experts in the field. The people with me were not as comfortable as I am because they carry some devices that occasionally make noise in their hands or on their backs. After fifteen or twenty steps, we needed to put on our gas masks. The plan was going to be executed without neglecting any details. I become the first one to break the rules. The gas mask bothers me a lot and makes it difficult to breathe. When I mention that I have to take off the mask, the other four people immediately say the same thing and remove their masks. Only one person, also to relieve tension a bit, says, "I don't want to die" and insists on walking with the mask, but it doesn't last long. As we are about to complete the first thousand meters, the increasing air flow begins to make itself felt, chilling us. While it's 40 degrees Celsius outside in August, we hadn't thought that we would have to wear our winter coats that we brought with us. We continued walking tightly dressed. Our minds were focused on each breath we took. There was little conversation. No one wanted to occupy their minds with anything else; we were only sniffing the air constantly. All the while, there was one thing that never left our minds, and I was afraid that this thought would turn into a nightmare as we got closer. I must have not realized that I was so influenced by what I heard from those who saw the 3700th meter where the incident took place. I feel as if what I heard, that dramatic scene, would welcome me a little later. Where we come to the last 500 meters, we come across a water source. In that section, an additional shoring was made against the ground looseness that the water would create and the dent was prevented. The workers put up a pipe to use some of the water as drinking water and gave it the air of a spring, albeit a primitive one.

We decided to take a short break by the water. One of our friends wanted to drink water with a plastic cup he took out of his bag. However, it was impossible to drink this water. Even touching it with a finger felt like being shocked. The water was colder than freezing point. Its flow prevented it from freezing. We couldn't drink the water and continued without waiting too long. The first thing I encountered was the mold I had made. The mold had been set up, and concrete had been poured, but it seemed like separating the mold from the concrete would be a bit difficult for me since it had exceeded the freezing time.

After freeing the mold from the concrete, I informed them to call the person who had used this mold in my absence to continue the work. It saddened me to hear that he had died on the spot while setting up the mold. Unfortunately, his nephew, whom he had brought along to train, shared the same fate. Whoever I asked, the answer I received was, "passed away". Since I was afraid of losing my mind if I stayed here, I finished my work as soon as possible and left on the same evening.

About one and a half to two months had passed since that incident. I was at the contractor company's office in Ankara, talking to a colleague when he said, "The report on the tunnel accident has been released, have you seen it?" He handed me a file he took out of his drawer. The report consisted of approximately a hundred pages. It was not possible to read and finish the file at that moment. So, I scanned the headings and read the subtitles that caught my attention. One headline caught my eye in the last section. The text summarized it as follows: "Based on the examination conducted, it was determined that the gas in question, which had an extremely high impact, caused sudden deaths. Even after losing its lethal property over time, if one remains in the environment for a long time, it is likely that some individuals may experience brain disorders in advanced ages...". The meaning of staying in the environment for a long time was not clear to me according to this report. I had only spent five to six hours there. But it is a fact that there were people who stayed in that environment, sniffing the air much more than I did. I currently have no way of reaching those people. It is not impossible, though difficult, to learn about the problems of these individuals. But what difference would it make to know the result of this investigation?

What am I doing? I realize that I am engaged in unnecessary efforts to learn what might have caused the incident in me. The incident has surrounded me at the moment. I know that a solution to completely eliminate its effect has not yet been found. However, I also know that scientists are working diligently to achieve that goal.

Therefore, I am convinced that I should focus my diminishing energy on this issue, thinking about how I can reduce the impact of the incident and improve my quality of life.

Fourth Battery

About two and a half years ago (2019), I made an appointment at the usual hospital for the replacement of my 4th battery. I stayed in the hospital a few days. I exchanged greetings with the doctor and caretakers I had met before. Some of the doctors had been promoted, while others had gone to serve in another part of the country. The head of the clinic became the Chief Physician. And here I am, completing the puzzle as a patient. Everything is going very well. I feel a little annoyed by their treatment of me as "one of them." Later, I apologize for being upset. I am assigned to the clinic's best and the only patient bed. Routine tests and examinations begin. Most of them are completed in one day.

The next day, I am reminded of my appointment with the psychologist. Half an hour later, the veteran caretaker comes pushing a wheelchair from the other end of the corridor. He stops in front of me. With a swift and graceful movement, he turns the wheelchair around its axis, bringing it to the most accessible position. And not only that, he finishes the ceremony with a royal salute. When my wife offers to push the wheelchair, he refuses and doesn't forget to compliment her.

"Would I ever send the most loyal customer of our hospital on foot?"

We continue the conversation along the way and arrive at the door of the psychologist's office. Our friendly attendant informs them that we have entered and leaves the room after placing the file he's holding. Upon our insistence, he hands over the wheelchair to my wife.

First, I underwent a test that I later understood was meant to measure my attention. They put on a pair of headphones. I heard a periodic beep sound, and occasionally, a different sound accompanied it. Every time I heard that sound, I had to press the button placed under my finger. Believing that I passed this test successfully, I was told that another test needed to be done before leaving the room. The psychologist is a young man in his 30s. There is no one else in the room. There couldn't be, because the room is so small and windowless, almost like a pantry. No one can stay in this room for more than ten minutes. If this man were to sit here for hours, it would indicate that he is mentally ill. I entered the room with my wife.

He handed me a book consisting of a series of shapes. He asked ten questions, such as completing the fourth shape by looking at three shapes placed side by side. Then he repeated ten two-digit numbers in a random order. Later, he asked me to repeat those numbers. I couldn't remember the last number on the first try. He repeated the same numbers once again. This time, I didn't make a mistake. He said that I had ten attempts and that I succeeded on my second try.

Later, he turned to my wife and asked her to leave us alone for two minutes. When my wife left the room, he asked me a very personal question about my sex life. When the question was asked without hiding behind words, I answered it honestly.

My session with the psychologist was over. Everything was ready to remove my old battery and replace it with a new one. After the tests, my wife and I went to the cafeteria to have something to drink. Just as we placed our orders, a phone call came in. It turned out that there were doctors waiting for us in our room. We hurriedly went to the room without even being able to enjoy our tea.

It was not a usual sight. Three young doctors, each holding a file with the word "Dr." embroidered on the pocket of their white uniforms, were waiting for me. This is a research hospital, and these young doctors have graduated and want to specialize in PD. An extraordinary case that caught their attention is reflected on their computer screens. That's why they find this fifteen-year PD patient worthy of examination. I tried to assist the research doctors until the day I was discharged from the hospital. Even while preparing my suitcases, I had to reject the request for an interview from a young doctor in the rush. Another specialist doctor in the same hospital had stated that due to the strong structure of the brain, it is very difficult for the disease to overcome the brain. Today, despite being a PD patient for 23 years, I could drive a car for 5 hours without any difficulty. What else can I do?

This year marks the 23th year of PH in my body. (This part was written in 2020). I have no idea how much of my 4th battery has been used. Some days, I open and close it about 4-5 times during the day. The previous batteries lasted about three and a half years because they were constantly running. During the assembly of this last battery, I experienced an unusual event, or rather a short sketch of dark humour.

I could tell from the sound of the wheels, which have run out of oil, that my famous caregiver is approaching with a stretcher instead of a wheelchair. He stops in front of the room, doing his usual turn.

"Come on gentlemen, the surgery shuttle is leaving. Those who miss it can take the Zincirlikuyu shuttle." What you need to know here is that Zincirlikuyu is the name of a famous cemetery in Istanbul.

I put on the surgical gown and lay down on the stretcher. We took a long journey. I was used to it. Hospital buildings usually have underground connections to each other. The operating room is on the top floor of the opposite building. By opposite building, I don't mean across the street. It's a bird's-eye distance, close to a hundred meters. We change three elevators. Finally, we arrive. My operation is a simple surgical operation. Despite that, the shaking on the way back causes discomfort. I think, for a patient coming out of a heart surgery or a surgery that cannot tolerate shaking, it cannot be said that there is no possibility of losing them during this journey.

I lie down on the operating table by changing three elevators and a rail system. The team, dressed in green, with an average age of 35, is taking it slow. I wait on the table like a sacrificial lamb. The truth comes out when I eavesdrop on their phone conversations. It turns out that the young representative of the company selling our battery got stuck in traffic, and everyone is waiting for him. They asked me if I wanted to get up. I said I was fine and just asked for a pillow. They must have noticed that I was a little cold because they also brought a blanket. Even if you're not sleep deprived, when you lie down all the time, sleep comes. While the team was chatting, I was hit by a tremendous sleep. Just in time, the new employee of my battery company showed up. The chief or president of the surgical team, or whatever they call her, is a young and beautiful woman. She looks like early 20s, but she has an air as if she is older than everyone there. She doesn't let herself be overwhelmed by the work she does despite her young age. She manages the necessary discipline not by yelling and shouting but by making confident decisions and leading the team with a management greyhound. She also doesn't forget to make measured jokes compressed into a good management description. Even just passing off her own joke without laughing becomes part of the quality.

She doesn't neglect to playfully brush off the battery representative. Since getting stuck in traffic is such a classic excuse for being late, he can't escape being scolded. The young representative is already excited because he has just started, so I felt like saying "don't be hard on him". My fear was that it wasn't the time or place to demoralize this young man, who was going to attend surgery a little later, and make the connections of the device.

The operation began. When I woke up, I found myself in my room, trying to figure out where exactly I was on the famous journey between the room and the operating room. I had finally received my new battery.

Hospitals and Voters

I started this book two years ago. During the past year, I chose to observe the illness on my body without writing anything. It is currently June 2021. We are experiencing a year where summer is late, or rather, it hasn't arrived yet. I don't refer to it as summer if I can't sit on the balcony in a t-shirt. Rain has a mocking attitude, as if asking, "Should I rain every three days or not?". One moment, we suddenly find ourselves in summer without experiencing the magnificent scent of spring, without picking daisies or watching butterflies dance. Currently, we can transition from winter to summer at any moment.

If a Parkinson's patient is asked to choose between the summer season and the winter season, they would ponder for a moment and choose the summer season. Of course, this preference varies depending on the environment the patient is in. Financial power determines that this preference is not an absolute truth. If a PH patient lacks financial comfort, it becomes more difficult for them to find physical comfort. It is certain that the absence of the comfortable and happy environments needed by a PD patient negatively affects the progression of their disease.

In our country, the political party and its supporters who have been in power for the past twenty years realized the extent of their power 3-5 years after coming into power. Finding themselves in the corn warehouse that a hungry chicken dreams of bewilders the majority from the voters to the leader. If one good deed is done, four corruptions are committed. This ratio is rapidly increasing day by day. As for the present, corruption fueled by the intoxication of public power, not just an economic downturn, has pushed the country off track. Some of the aware public are filled with concern. As long as the narrow-minded perspective of the ruling party, fixated on a single direction with blinders, does not change, it seems difficult for this order to change.

The actions of this government, which has left its mark on the past twenty years, are exaggerated with lies. During this time, voters who couldn't conceive of what could be achieved with this budget saw the actions as extraordinary achievements. The necessary actions by the government were adorned, further narrowing the tunnel vision of the uneducated masses.

To say that there have been no right actions apart from the routine services of this government that has been in power for so many years would not be in line with an objective perspective. Perhaps the only positive service that has been done is in the field of healthcare. Taking a brief look at the past, let's start with hospitals. The variety of hospitals serving different segments such as state hospitals, insurance hospitals, private hospitals of public institutions, and fully private hospitals has been eliminated. Thus, while state hospitals remained empty or less crowded, getting an appointment at an insurance hospital was considered a miracle. If the examination time in a small room exceeded three minutes, negative murmurs would start from outside.

Today, thanks to the development of communication systems, patients can make appointments online and even choose their doctors.

Another revolutionary achievement in the healthcare sector was the opening of private hospitals to the public for a contribution fee. These and a few other significant changes have been the success of this government in favor of the people. However, while doing all this, the fact that they have worked a thousand times more for the people and the dimensions of these corruptions have threatened the public assets of the Republic of Turkey, casting a shadow over the government's success in the healthcare system. The fanatic group of supporters of the ruling party openly expressing the logic of "they steal but they work" has given courage to the party members who were already inclined towards theft. The situation has gotten out of hand. People on the streets who are not worth greeting are being appointed as administrators in public institutions. Most of the graduates from imam hatip schools (vocational schools where students were to be trained as preachers and ministers or prepared for higher education) who are members of the ruling party are in a race to sink these institutions that they cannot manage. Although the system looks very good, when the majority of the people running this system are of imam origin, it becomes inevitable for the results to be negative.

University hospitals can also be added to this list. According to the old system, university hospitals were providing services to insured patients in return for a contribution fee from the beginning. According to the recent practice, the cost of the examination or treatment is covered by the Social Security Institution according to the protocol made with the institution. Some university hospitals charge extra fees to patients, especially when it is necessary to apply imported devices due to the nature of the disease, claiming that the amount paid by the state or the social security institution is insufficient. I experienced this reality during my recent battery replacement.

Ankara is far away, so we started researching to find a hospital in our city where the battery replacement could be done. We met with a doctor who performs this procedure. We were informed that an additional 7-8 thousand lira (~1,400 USD at the time) was required, so I applied to the hospital in Ankara again for the battery replacement. The battery I mentioned is the one I am currently carrying, and I control the on-off function myself.

DBS and Personal Life

In recent days, most of my friends with PD have been messaging me, seeking information about the battery. In the upcoming chapters of my book, I mainly want to talk about DBS treatment and its effects on me.

As I mentioned at the beginning of the book, PD varies from person to person. It is known as the shaking disease, and those who are not familiar with the disease may not be aware of its symptoms other than shaking. Tremors, freezing, excessive slowness of movement, difficulty in walking, and imbalance are some of the symptoms. Not all of these symptoms appear together, but all the other symptoms are hidden within these signs and can occur at any moment depending on the medication you are taking.

I want to talk about my daily life, specifically the part related to PD. I'm talking about a patient who has been diagnosed with Parkinson's disease for about 26 years, experienced ups and downs during this period, was bedridden at one point, and couldn't walk at another. Today, as I am writing this, the time is 2:10 AM. I feel as tired as anyone who is awake at this hour. I can foresee enduring another half an hour. Then I turn on the battery, which is currently off. I place it within easy reach of my bed, considering that I may not be able to get up for a bathroom break during the night. I believe that urinary incontinence is a common occurrence among patients. That's why I'm always cautious.

I must fall asleep within ten minutes of lying in bed. If I can't achieve that, I may face some difficulties the next day. With regular sleep and a refreshed mind, as soon as I open my eyes in the morning, I can predict how my day will go. Actually, staying up until this hour is a big mistake, and I acknowledge that.

...

Good morning, friends. If I went to bed late last night and I'm up at this hour (8:30 AM), it means I'm feeling good. I spent about five hours asleep. Five hours of quality sleep is sufficient for me. I feel the need to explain in case you've noticed. When I told my doctor that I use the battery in an on-off manner, he said, "That's possible. For example, you should turn it off at night." On the contrary, if I don't turn on the battery, muscle stiffness, albeit to a lesser extent, involuntary movements, and difficulty in turning left and right hinder my sleep. The most bothersome symptom is the cramping of my feet.

The first thing I do when I wake up in the morning is to take the first dose of the day's medication. I take a slightly higher dose (200mg) than the dose I take during the day (150mg).

While consuming protein-rich foods during breakfast, I am extremely measured. There are so many things that contain protein, and I think violating the rules by consuming protein is at the top of the list. It has been found that patients who have undergone DBS surgery using brain implants should avoid taking excessive amounts of vitamins. Excessive protein intake and vitamin supplements can cause inflammation around the areas where the metal diodes (a very special metal, of course) implanted in the brain come into contact due to compatibility issues with these diodes. You're right. I don't fully understand it either. What I need to understand is that I shouldn't be having too much vitamins and protein.

During dinner, I sit with the battery on. Once I finish eating, I get up from the table and immediately switch to the off mode, meaning the battery is turned off. Since the medication has started to take effect, having both the battery and the medication active greatly contributes to freezing.

By the way, you should take good care of the battery remote control in your hand. It is better to avoid movements that can cause it to fall, collide, or be mishandled. It has an exorbitant price.

The patient should perform the switch of the battery themselves. The power settings of the battery should be made by your doctor. You can see the device that makes this power setting only during the doctor's examination or during the examination about the battery settings. This setting is very important. The doctor expects the result from the patient after each new adjustment. When the patient is in the best condition, that setting registers on the device.

I want to emphasize once again that this doesn't apply to every patient. I am personally sure that the battery must be used in the on-off manner. The details, timing, whether the on-off times are correct or not, and the implementation of this method are left to my fellow Parkinson's patients who have undergone brain implant surgery and their supportive family members who help them in every aspect.

When we talk about family members, we usually think of one of the relatives. PD progresses insidiously, and the most intense stage coincides with the elderly period. It is necessary to start preparing for this stage in advance. The most important preparation is to have a person, a close friend, whom the patient can rely on. We never know what the future holds. Even when one has full confidence in their spouses/partners, it's still beneficial to have a backup plan.

Balance and imbalance are another troublesome symptom of PD. Sometimes, a leaf of a tree is enough to maintain balance. Holding onto something or someone's arm while walking helps prevent loss of balance. Another difficulty is trying to walk with short steps. It gives the feeling that someone is pulling from the front. It has been observed that when attempting to walk unsupported and unassisted, my steps become almost 10 cm or less.

I cannot skip telling an anecdote about walking with short steps. During a bus journey from Bursa to Ankara, our bus took a break at a roadside rest area. Unfortunately, the break time coincided with my off position. This was unlucky because I needed to use the restroom, and if I had to walk to the restroom alone, I would have missed the bus. I got off the bus, and the first person I encountered was a gas station attendant. When he saw me, he immediately came up to me and said,

"Brother, let me help you."

I told him the same thing I always tell people who try to assist me by holding onto my arm. I said,

"It's easier if you extend your arm for me to hold onto instead of holding onto my arm."

Despite the difficult walk with short steps, I managed to fulfill my needs and returned to the bus in the same way. I didn't let go of his arm until we reached the bus door. I was about to thank him and leave when the young attendant asked a surprising question, to which I responded with a bewildered "no." I didn't have time to explain. The question he asked was,

"Brother, are you blind from birth?"

...

As I mentioned before, three months after the brain implant surgery, I started experiencing speech difficulties, which led me to quit a commitment I had made before even starting it. For four years, I couldn't speak. It was a very distressing four years. I was practically mute. I don't think I can achieve speaking by trying hard. During my efforts in this regard, I am aware that I put the person in front of me in a difficult position when I focus my energy and brain and ask a question, and their reaction sometimes annoys me. Even though they didn't understand the question, they pretend they did and try to dismiss it with a yes or a nod. I insist and tell them that I know they didn't understand and ask why they didn't ask again, but some still pretend they understood. On the other hand, there are people who persistently try to understand and, if necessary, bring their ear closer and ask me to repeat the question or what I was trying to say until they understand. I always appreciate that.

Because the difficulty to speak, or rather the problem of not being able to communicate at all sometimes, is very different from other troubles. It is impossible to understand and explain this scourge without experiencing it. There have been times when I have reached the point of going crazy because of this.

I can see imagine you are hesitant about the brain implant battery now. It is possible to say that the brain implant surgery is not an easy procedure. It is a difficult and costly operation. Incompatibility between the battery and the body can cause significant problems. Additionally, the battery has an active lifespan that varies between three and a half to five years, depending on usage. Although removing the battery and replacing it seems like a simple operation every four years, in the end, you will need to spend at least a week in the hospital. During this time, you will undergo surgery under anesthesia.

Another event that seems negative to me is that the operation is always performed from the same place, even the same spot. I haven't heard from doctors that it has any harm to the body, but I haven't heard that it doesn't either. For the next battery replacement, I am determined to use an externally rechargeable battery. I haven't done the research yet. According to the hearsay information I gathered, a rechargeable battery that lasts for a week during full usage is installed. The battery is charged for two hours every day of the week. Although I am not able to include detailed information about the latest developments around it, not requiring another surgery for battery replacement alone can be a preference. I recommend readers who consider the operation to do their research about this.

When I was in the hospital in Ankara, I met many patients in the neurology department. A patient in his 50s caught my attention. His eyelids wouldn't open. He wasn't blind. We were talking. When he wanted to see, he would lift his eyelid with his finger, and when he finished, his eyelid would drop on its own. He wants to show me a note he wrote on his phone. I read it.

"12 years ago, one morning, I realized that I was like this."

Why did I tell this story? At occasions I haven't figured out yet, my eyelids drop, and I struggle to open them. I noticed that this happens when the battery is off. When I turn the battery "on," meaning when it's active, my eyes and eyelids return to normal. For now, I'm trying to understand the reason behind this incident.

Falls

My knee joints are on the verge of rebellion. Falling is one of the most frequent complaints lately. Depending on the severity of the fall, each fall gradually shortens the lifespan of my knees.

The period with intense falling coincides with the time when the effect of the medication is fully active and the battery has not yet been turned off. Falls occur as a result of freezing and decrease to a level where disabling the battery doesn't have much effect.

I can say that I'm fascinated by my wife's description of my illness. She says, "He can't walk but can climb stairs, he can't walk but can drive a car, he can't walk but can run." The fear of falling is a very disturbing feeling. Trying not to fall while walking unsupported alone sometimes leads to falls. Although not always, when falling becomes inevitable, I have the opportunity to think about how I can fall in the least harmful way. I don't have time to stop, calm down, and focus on taking that last step. During that time, vehicles approaching rapidly come dangerously close to hitting me. They barely miss me. It's usually more advantageous to stay in the middle of the road rather than being one step away from the finish line. Because when I'm in the middle, vehicles notice me or I can make a gesture to make them stop. This incident has made me quite knowledgeable about the psychological states of drivers. Some people think that when they drive a car, they can control the world. Those who act like monsters behind the wheel realize that they are actually nothing when they get out of the car. Imagine a driver noticing my unique way of walking due to my illness, stopping at least ten meters away, turning off the car, and signaling for me to stay calm. Some of the vehicles behind also notice the situation and wait in the same way, while others honk as much as they can. At that moment, unnecessary panic starts within me. I cause this scene, but why? The reason behind all the honking, the arguments that sometimes turn into fights between the ones in front and the ones behind, is me. As I think about these, my anxiety increases even more, and all parts of my body except my feet start making forward movements. The feet and the body can't seem to agree, and the connection is severed, meaning I fall. I have to protect my knees because both of them have filled their quota, and now the hands and palms have taken over the task of making initial contact with the ground. Suddenly, I realize that the honking has stopped. Two strong hands under my armpits lift me off the ground, and I am standing again. There is silence among the waiting vehicles. Those who caused a commotion with their honking are now buried in silence. They wait for the road to clear with a half-embarrassed demeanor. The two people who lifted me off the ground try to move me aside by lifting my feet this time. This wasn't so easy. After all, I weighed around a hundred kilograms. I thought it was time for me to intervene and said to my friends, "Hold on a second, gentlemen. You don't need to drag me. One person on my right side can just hold my arm in a supportive manner, that's enough for me." They are doing exactly what I said, and I cross the street as if the person they just lifted from the previous spot wasn't me, taking small steps. I thank my friends and continue on my way. They are too shocked to respond to my gratitude, and amidst their bewildered looks, I feel the joy of surviving another falling incident unharmed.

While telling this example, I might not have emphasized it enough. Freezing, which is not as troublesome as it sounds, is a significant and bothersome symptom of PD. The patient's helper, spouse, friend, partner, or whoever is there for them; in such situations, simply extending their arm without exerting force will be sufficient. Another solution is to ask the patient themselves what they need to do at that moment.

Dreams

I can't say I used to dream very often before PD. I would forget the dream by morning. I never had the urge to shout, scream, or get out of bed while being caught up in the atmosphere of the dream. After DBS surgery, I started having a lot of dreams. And boy, did they start! I mean, I want to say it was like colorful Turkish cinema in cinemascope. Magnificent scenarios, clear and uninterrupted visuals... They were all present in my dreams.

If I had the chance to choose between my old dreams and my new dreams, I wouldn't hesitate for a minute. Despite the image quality of my new dreams, I would never trade my old dreams. Because when watching a dream or playing a role in it, I would try to perform the same movements. The voiceover is extremely perfect, but in the dreams where I play the leading role, my voice that doesn't come out when I'm awake grates on my ears in my dreams. I am awakened by my wife. We exchange a few words. Then I go back to sleep. It's very interesting... I continue from where I left off. The incident doesn't end with shouting.

And if there is a scene of violence at that moment, and if I am in that scene...

...

In one of my dreams, I had to jump off a trampoline as part of my role. I jumped, but I couldn't dive into the water. I opened my eyes with a tremendous headache. My wife and little son were changing the position of the ice pack they had placed on my head.

"What happened to me?" I asked.

My wife replied, "You should ask yourself. Your son says he saw you flying in the air. Where were you going?"

"I was jumping into the pool. Where is the pool? Where am I? Oh my God, I jumped into an empty pool. How could I not see that the pool was empty?"

When I jumped off the trampoline, aiming for the water pool, and finding it empty, I had thrown myself with all my strength against the opposite wall. After a week of physical therapy, my pain subsided, and I continued to live with PD, successfully avoiding another major danger.

Animals

I believe there is a strange and interesting relationship between animals and Parkinson's patients. In fact, I was not an animal lover. I even used to engage in winter hunting. On a cold and snowy winter day, I dress warmly and take the hunting rifle to go for a walk. There are plenty of blackbirds around. It's evident that they are hungry because everything is covered in snow. They fly around in a frenzy, searching for food. Some of them, exhausted from their search, hang on a tree branch, waiting to freeze to death. I choose one of them and pull the trigger. It falls to the ground. I reach it quickly as the snow allows. I realize in my palm that it's not dead yet. But I think it only has a few minutes to live. At that moment, we make eye contact. These eyes that are about to close forever had saved their last gaze to impress me. They were speaking to me, as if they were saying something. Those eyes were like they were talking. They were telling me something I would never forget in my life.

"You think you saved me by shooting me because I was dying of hunger. I don't want two grains of wheat from you to save me. If you had let me peacefully freeze and die without suffering, that would have been better. Now you're going to cook and eat me. You will satisfy your hunger by eating a starving bird. Do you know that you and other humans... are more savage and predatory than some animals you call predators?"

These were his final words. He slowly closed his eyes. The faint trembling that indicated signs of life ceased, and his furry body grew colder in my palm. A handful of bird taught me such a lesson that I started experiencing interesting feelings towards animals since that day.

To live with him and keep him alive, we adopted Mia. She was a stray cat, but now she brings joy to our home. I hadn't wanted to adopt a cat before she came. Because I preferred dogs. But I thought that having a dog required a house with a garden.

Mia, on the other hand, lives in our home as one of us. We adjust everything according to her. She took away our family's freedom. Despite everything, we love her very much.

About two years after the DBS surgery. Despite the battery, I could not be considered very well. I still had walking difficulties and speech problems. During that time, I met with friends almost every day in a garden operated by an association that rented it from the municipality, located 500 meters away from my home. Its proximity to my house was an advantage for me, as it was a healthier and more suitable place than the café. Its regulars were not only humans.

In my opinion, the true owners of the garden were them. The locals living nearby said that they were born and raised there. There were four of them. Their peaceful nature was evident from their good relationship with each other. We know that dogs have certain abilities that modern technology cannot achieve. Their highly developed sense of smell allows them to detect things that even the most advanced detectors cannot. In addition to that, they have a sense of adoption and protection, which they proved to me by experiencing it.

The time had come to return from the garden where I went almost every day. One of the dogs, resembling a shepherd dog, caught my attention. It was sitting in front of me right now, waiting in its classic posture. I remember the previous day. It had come and sat in the same place at the same time. Moreover, yesterday, it seemed like it was escorting me to the doorstep of my house without breaking a ten-meter distance between us. Today, the same thing happened again. I got up from the table, ready to go home. After saying goodbye to my friends, I set off on the road. I glanced back. When I reached halfway and looked back, I couldn't believe my eyes. I had no doubt that this animal was an extraordinary creature. When it saw me stopping, it also stopped and turned away as if it didn't recognize me. Respecting it may be seen as funny by many people. But no matter what anyone says, I respect these creatures. I believe that they have the ability to recognize the disease. There are also dog breeds suitable for home conditions. I highly recommend having a dog that is smarter and has a stronger sense of adoption than others.

Final

As a Parkinson's patient for over 20 years, I have shared with you the issues that I have personally observed and felt, and only the outcomes that have affected me positively or negatively. I want to emphasize that I have no intention of directing anyone. Accordingly, I am listing the elements of my struggle with Parkinson's disease in order of importance as follows:

1. DBS: The brain battery surgery had a 30-35% positive effect on me. Its most significant effect was relieving the stiffness in my legs.

2. Sleep: The second most important factor after the battery. At least 6 hours of quality and uninterrupted sleep per day.

3. Nutrition: Try getting up from the table without feeling full. After seeing the results, even if you want to eat more, you won't be able to. Certain things will happen naturally. I achieved results by doing so because it was necessary for the medication to take effect immediately. Medications are effective when taken on an empty stomach. Since I take 6 doses a day, I don't have time to stay hungry. That's why I

settle for half a portion. Focus on vegetable dishes, especially olive oil broccoli and cauliflower salad, and you can consume all vegetables except broad beans. The recommendation of fiber-rich foods for constipation is useless. Vegetables, vegetables, vegetables. But in season if possible.

4. Water: One glass of quality water for each dose of medication. I don't recommend it, I urge you to do it. If you can't do this, neither the medication nor anything else will work. The usual consequence of not doing this is kidney failure.

5. Sports: I enjoy sports as a spectator. I find excessive sports unnecessary. I am a bit lazy in this regard. So it would be more accurate not to take advice from me.

6. Smoking and alcohol: Actually, these two should be separated. There have been many times when I could only cross the street after lighting my cigarette and taking a breath. As for alcohol, it takes back the pleasure it gives when consumed the next day, multiplied by several times.

7. Environment: PD patients need a peaceful environment just like anyone else, but they need it twice as much.

With best wishes for a speedy recovery to all Parkinson's patients.

The end.